The Ultimate Guide to Essential Oils

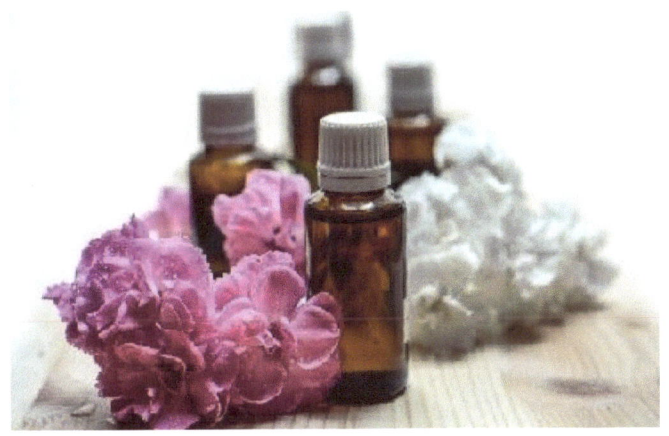

Written By Alicia Phillips

The Writer of The Happy Hippie

About the Author

Hello my Happy Hippies!

My name is Alicia Phillips, I am a 22 year old who lives in a small suburban town outside of Philadelphia.

I am the writer of The Happy Hippie and starting this blog has changed my life. Not only am I happy, but I am finding success helping others as well.

One way I have managed to keep calm during this exciting, but sometimes stressful adventure is by using my essential oils ALL. THE. TIME!

Honestly, I never thought I would get into the concept of essential oils, but I decided to dive in and now, they are doing some amazing things.

What amazing things? I am sure you are asking that.

Well, when I was 18, I was diagnosed with severe anxiety disorder. It was the scariest thing that ever happened to me because I felt like I had lost control of my mind completely.

I took medication for four years. At the end of those four years, I truly started feeling so much better. So I made the crazy decision to get off my medicine. I did not want to have to rely on it any longer. I thought this was going to be super easy and painless. Wrong, because while I was weening off of it, I felt like I was losing my mind, I felt like I was going to pass out 24/7 and I was extremely irritable. It was horrible.

With about two weeks left of weening off my medication, I decided to try some essential oils. I wanted a natural remedy to replace my medication, and I figured this moment was as good as any other, if not better since I was already losing it.

So I purchased some starter oils and a diffuser, and suddenly, my life completely changed.

I know that sounds super cliche but it is so true, my life changed.

I was ecstatic, I now had a natural way to cope with my anxiety. I had found a healthy replacement to my medication.

This was pretty much the best discovery I had ever made and I am constantly using my oils!

So take the dive with me and come learn about the amazing benefits these oils have in store for you!

Intro to the Oils
Because what are they anyway?

I guess this would be a good place to start, right?

Essential oils are natural plant extracts that are turned into liquid. They are 100% natural and safe for your body and offer many health benefits.

That is actually the cool thing about these oils because every one offers something different.

There are also multiple ways you can use them.

My favorite way is to blend a few in my diffuser. My diffuser then extracts a constant mist into the air. As I breathe in, I am breathing in the oils and all of their aromatherapy affects. It is so calming.

I also have a necklace that has a sponge in the middle. I take that sponge out of the necklace, apply a few drops of my favorite oil on it, and then I am constantly spelling the oil all day. This is especially great when you know you have a stressful day upon you. You are able to naturally relax all day. Aromatherapy is by far my favorite way to use my oils.

But, there are many more.

You can clean with them, add them to your water or food, use them for acne, athlete's foot, and stretch marks just to name a few.

Like I said, every oil has a different benefit.

You can pretty much just go throw out all of your toxic medications right now because essential oils are taking over and providing the same exact benefits in a natural way.

And this is just the start.

Lavender
It is only appropriate to start with the most popular oil out there, right?

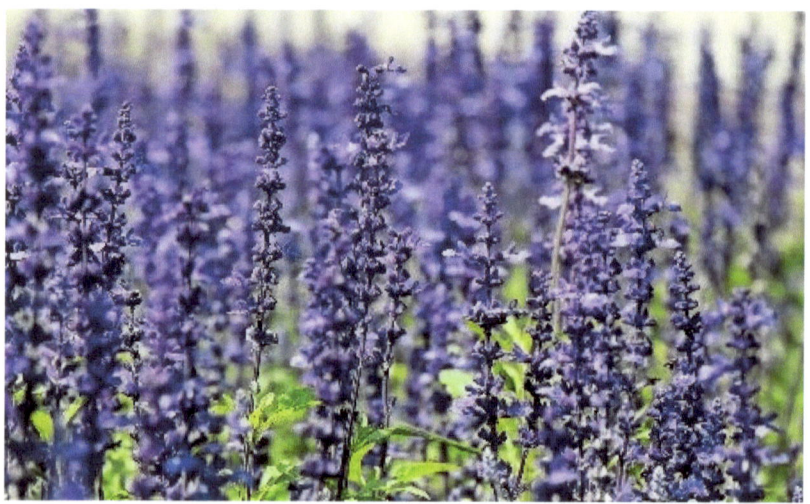

Lavender is one of the most popular oils out there and the benefits are amazing! This calming scent works wonders for your mind and body. A few of its benefits are:

• Skin irritation and Muscle Tension

• Reduces stress and anxiety

• Promotes healthy sleep habits

• Eases tension both physically and emotionally

• Helps reduce acne

• Helps remove wrinkles

• Prevents dandruff

• Reduces hair loss

• Reduces dark circles under eyes

Rose
The scent of romance

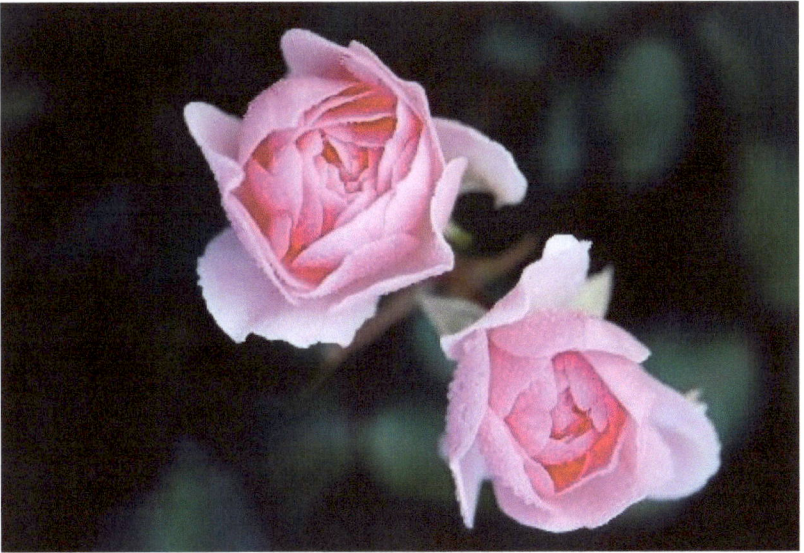

Rose, such a romantic and calming scent. Rose is much more rare, but the benefits it holds make it so worth finding.

- Natural Perfume

- Reduces stress and anxiety

- Helps fight grief, shock and depression

- Natural muscle relaxant

- Lowers inhibitions

- Boosts confidence

- Prevents infection in wounds
- Improves skin texture
- Natural laxative
- Purifies blood
- Prevents liver and stomach infection
- Helps prevent muscle cramps
- Strengthen gums
- Strengthens Hair roots
- Helps stimulate menstruation and boosts libido

Ylang Ylang
Let's get healthy

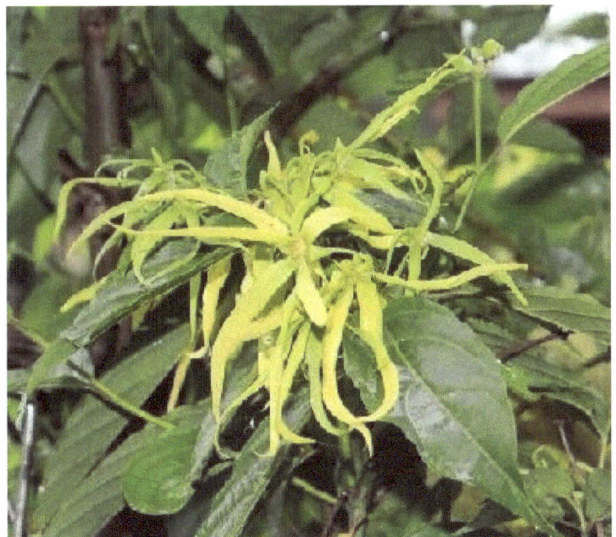

Even though it took my forever to learn how to pronounce, it has deemed itself to remain one of my all time favorite essential oils, and as always, the benefits show why.

- Regulates heartbeat
- Heals cardiac problems
- Increases blood flow
- Lifts mood (helps reduce stress, anxiety, and depression)
- Promotes healthy intentional function
- Relieves inflammation
- Helps balance hormones

- Promotes healthy skin and hair

Frankincense
Moving right along here...

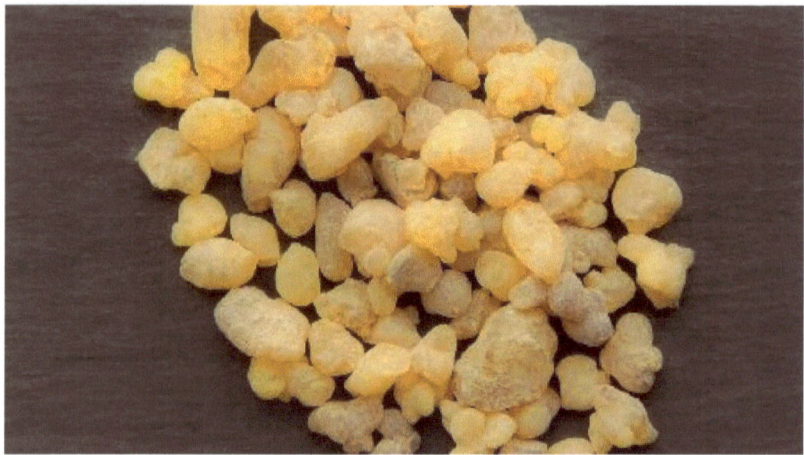

Frankincense is right up there with my favorite essential oils. It is such a unique scent, you really have to just try it out for yourself! And, as always, it comes with a ton of amazing benefits.

- Reduces anxiety and stress
- Reduces wrinkles
- Natural cold and flu prevention
- Immune system boost
- Promotes healthier and better sleep
- Natural home cleaner
- Helps indigestion
- Helps heal wounds and scars
- Regulates hormones

- Great for oral hygiene

Peppermint
That wonderful winter scent...

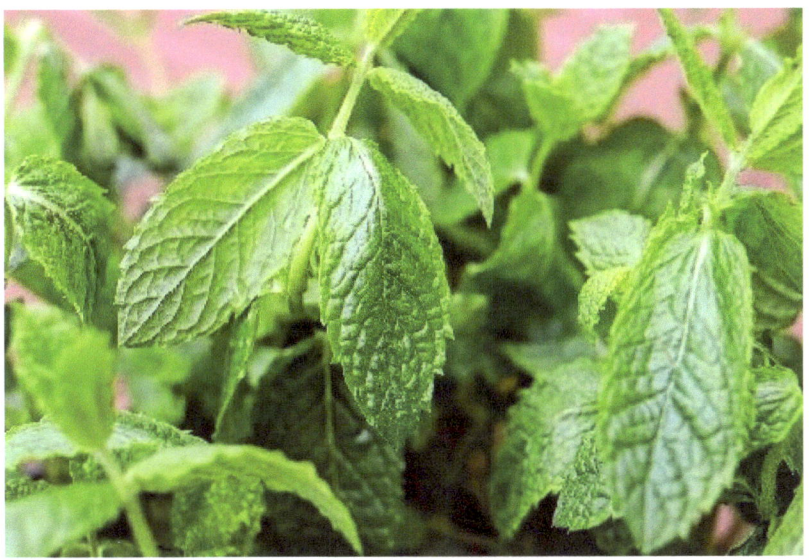

I use peppermint on a daily basis, I seriously love it that much! It helps me sleep so soundly and, especially when allergy season started, I blended it with lemon and lavender to create the perfect allergy blend. It was nice being able to actually breathe! But, of course, there are more benefits than just that!

- Muscle pain relief

- Sinus Relief

- Headache relief

- Reduces hunger cravings

- Joint relief

- Allergy relief
- Helps reduce fevers
- Acne treatment
- Skin health
- Natural bug repellant

Lemon
Let's get a little citrus in here

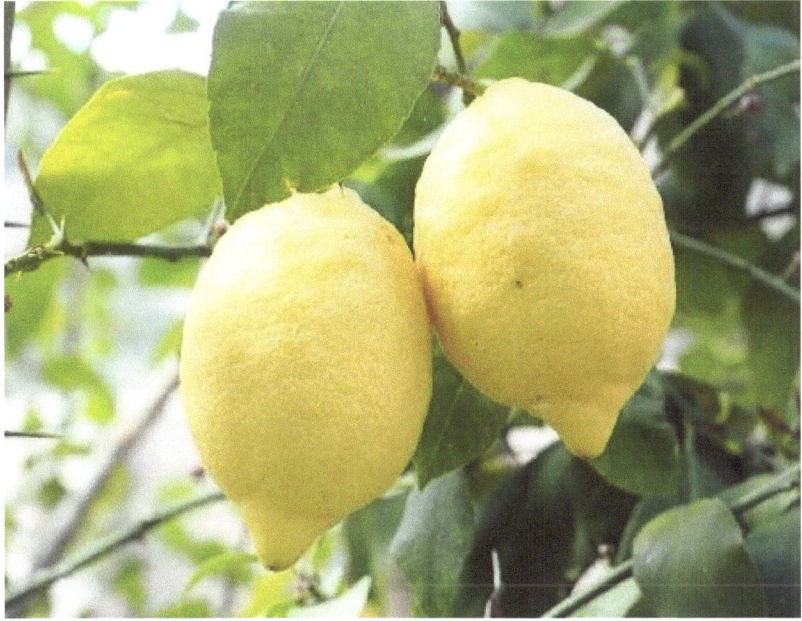

Lemon is one of my all time favorites! There is just something about the fresh aroma it puts off, and on top of that, it is stacked with benefits!

- Clears acne

- Antioxidant

- Anxiety

- Helps fight common colds

- Fever reducer

- Arthritis
- Lowers blood pressure
- Helps ease sore throat
- Disinfectant
- Fights food poisoning
- Helps with postpartum depression
- Relieves heartburn

Vetiver
A magical scent

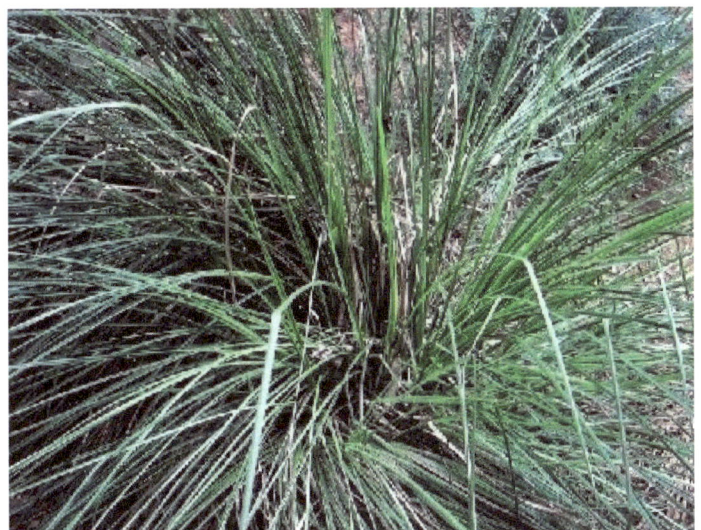

Vetiver is an all time favorite of many. Find out why!

- Anxiety

- Helps with sleep

- Aids depression

- Helps with ADD and hyperactivity

- Reduces fevers

- Eases nerves

- Reduces mestral cramps

- Reduces headaches

- Boosts energy
- Helps with focus
- Fights acne
- Helps with arthritis
- Fights wrinkles

Lime
Continuing with the citrus...

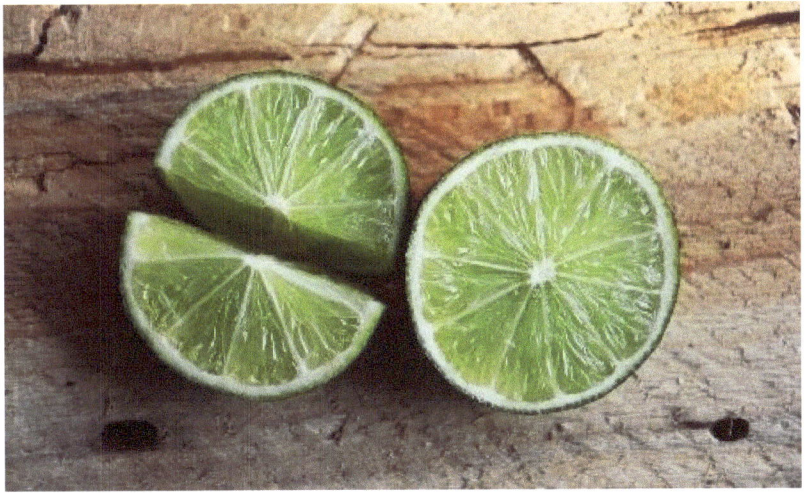

Along with lemon, lime helps keep things fresh! It is a familiar scent that is loved by many, with many benefits to love!

- Revitalizes skin

- Antiviral

- Lowers blood pressure

- Helps relieve sore throat

- Dissolves cellulite

- Water and air purification

- Helps with bacterial infections

- Antiseptic
- Soothes broken capillaries
- Restorative
- Good for cleaning children's skin
- Soothes insect bites
- Boosts immune system
- Encourages weight loss
- Fights depression

Melaleuca (Tea Tree Oil)
The first aid oil

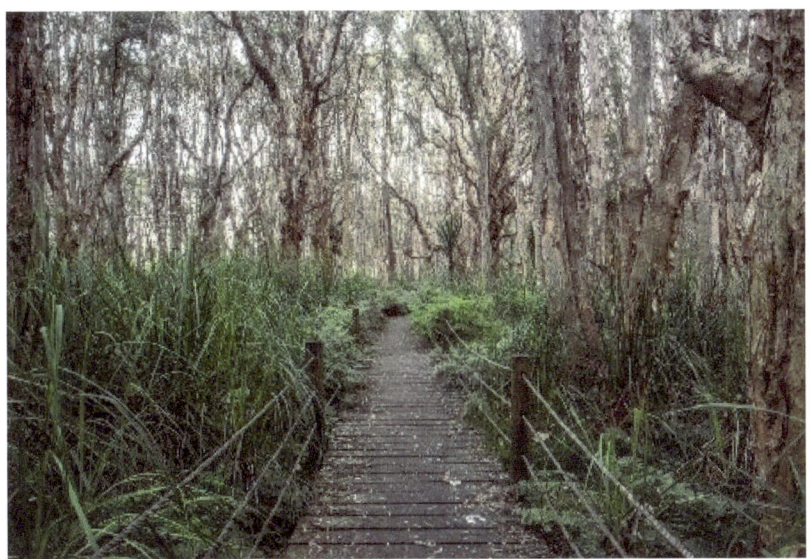

First aid in a bottle, but of course, it is also good for so much more!

- Cleans abrasions and cuts
- Fights acne
- Helps heal burns
- Fights ear infection
- Soothes rashes
- Fights sore throat
- Helps bad breath

- Fights bladder infection
- Fights head lice
- Soothes flea bites
- Removes mold
- Reduces inflammation
- Good for cleaning
- Fights ringworm
- Pest control
- Fights athletes foot
- Helps with chapped lips
- Fights dandruff
- Natural air freshener
- Helps with blisters

Oregano
This one is not only for the kitchen

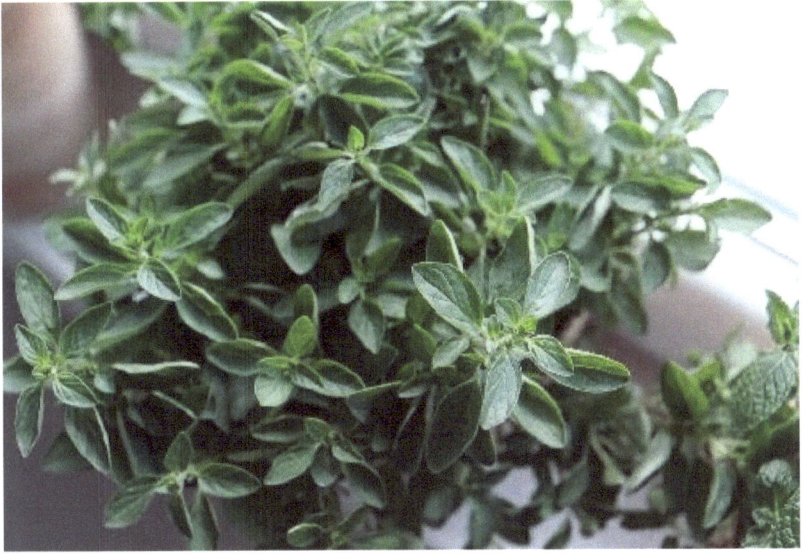

A classic spice in the kitchen, but its benefits as an oil can take this herb that much farther.

- Tick removal
- Anti-cancer
- Anti-fungal
- Antiviral
- Antibacterial
- Boost immunity
- Fights Allergies

- Fights inflammation
- Fights parasites
- Helps reduce warts
- Cold and flu remedy
- Fights mold
- Fights ulcers

Clary Sage
Even the name is gorgeous

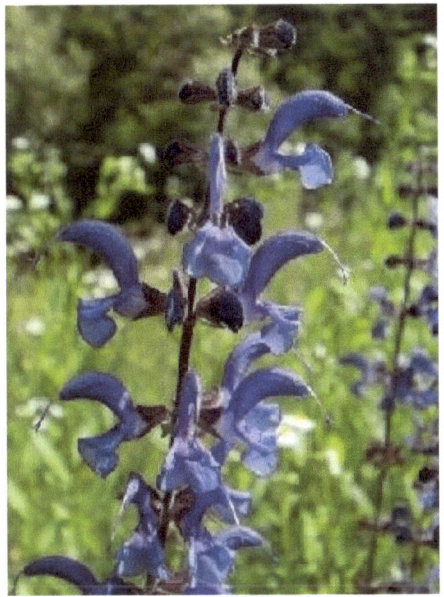

This beautiful plant smells as good as it looks. It also is packed with amazing perks.

- Relieves menstrual pain
- Supports hormonal balance
- Fights insomnia
- Increases circulation
- Stress reliever

- Reduces cholesterol
- Fights leukemia
- Kills bacteria
- Fights infection
- Calms the nervous system
- Improves memory
- Can promote relaxation during child birth
- Treats dandruff
- Stimulates hair growth
- Fights acne and oily skin
- Supports healthy digestive system
- Boosts libido

Lemongrass
Moving right along here

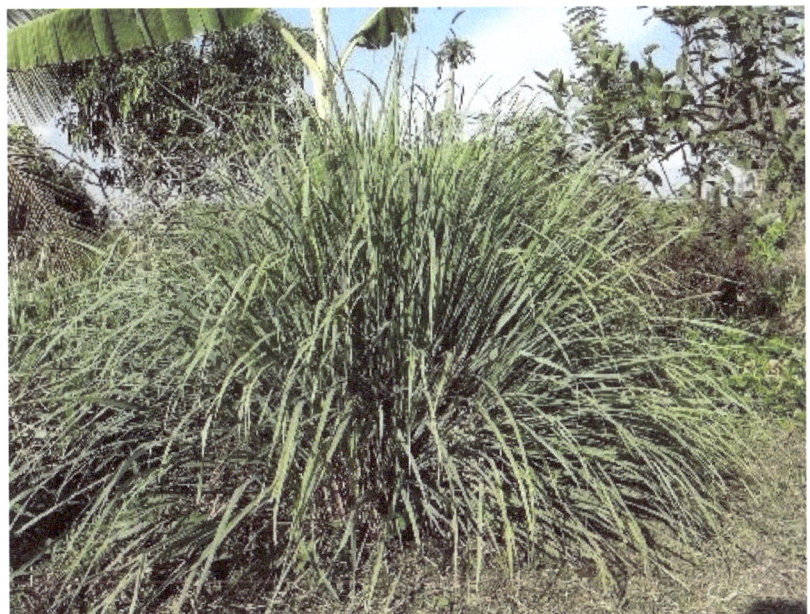

Once again, another oil that will not disappoint you!

- Natural deodorizer

- Promotes skin health

- Promotes hair health

- Stress reducer

- Aids sleep

- Natural bug repellant

- Muscle relaxer

- Headache relief

- Natural detox

- Stomach protector and Gastric Ulcer Cure

- Helps relieve nerve pain

- Helps with diarrhea

- Helps with carpal tunnel

- Soothes ligament pain

Eucalyptus
Let the soothing continue

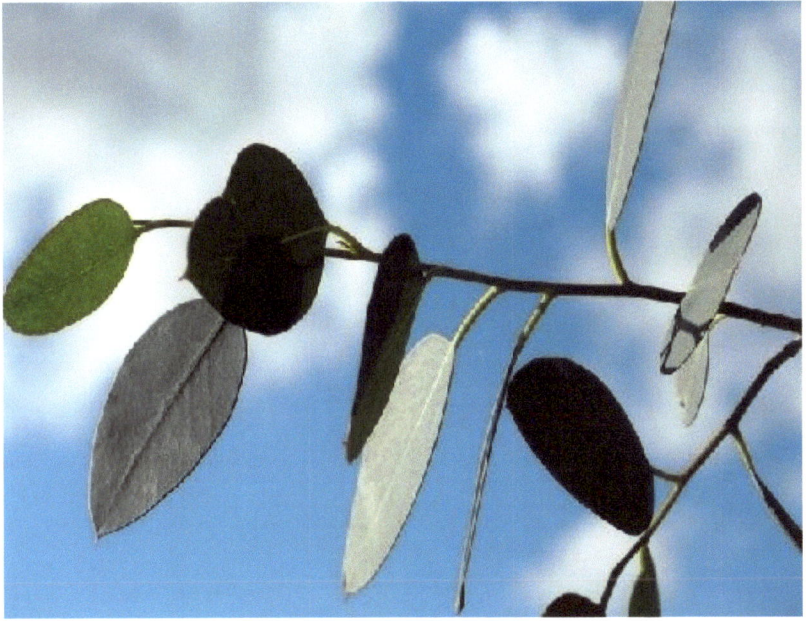

Another one of my favorites. Eucalyptus will not disappoint.

- Eases coughing
- Helps with asthma
- Fights congestion
- Fights respiratory issues
- Clears sinuses
- Fights allergies

- Fights bronchitis
- Fights pneumonia
- Soothes joint pain
- Reduces hot flashes
- Reduces fever
- Reduces headaches
- Fights the flu
- Boosts energy
- Reduces inflammation
- Fights shingles
- Fights kidney stones
- Soothes muscle pain

Helichrysum
This one does it all

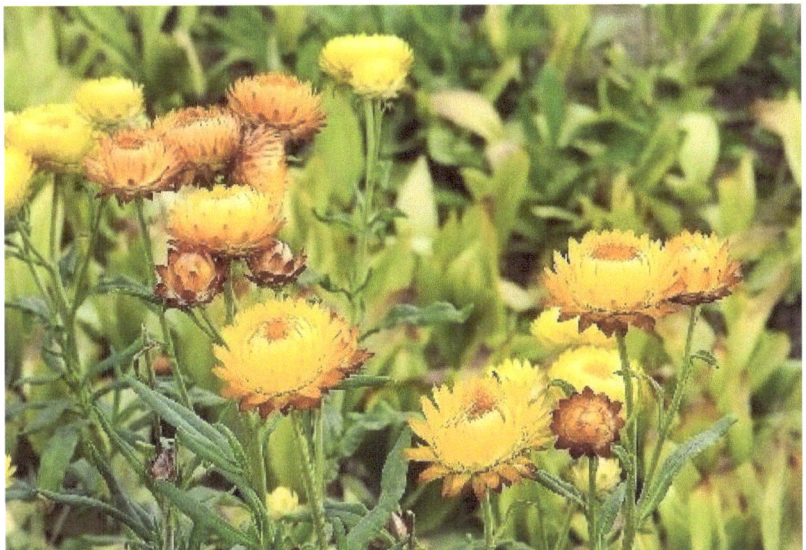

This one literally does it all, so basically you need it.

- Soothes arthritis pain

- Fights cold and flu

- Fights allergies

- Soothes sprains and strains

- Soothes muscle and tendon aches

- Reduces inflammation

- Fights asthma, tuberculosis, and whooping cough

- Fights acne
- Helps heal burns
- Good for wounds and rashes
- Increases circulation
- Fights bronchitis
- Soothes skin irritation
- Eases itching
- Helps with eczema and psoriasis
- Fights athlete's foot
- Helps heal bruises
- Reduces scarring
- Reduces wrinkles

Bergamot
Another anti-depressant, can medication just disappear now?

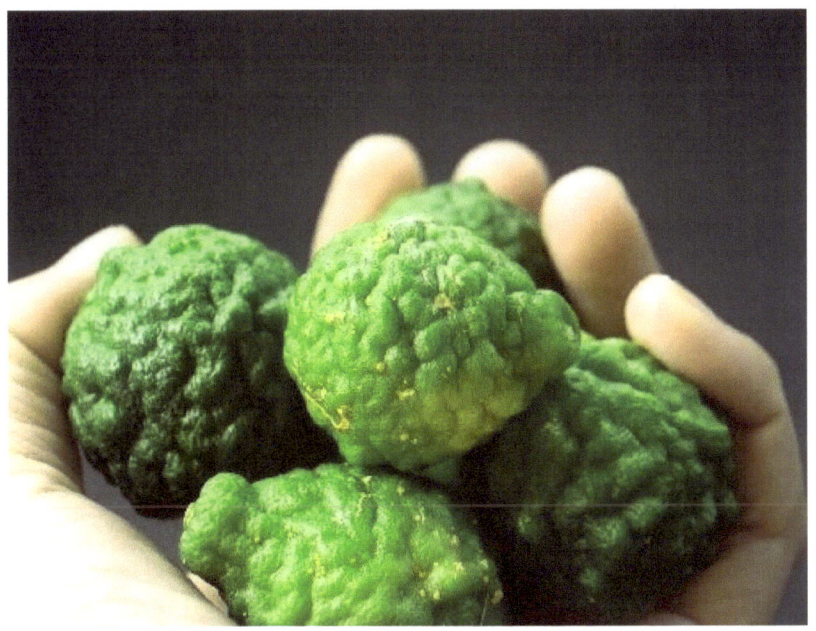

I am seriously so surprised I didn't learn about essential oils earlier, I mean, the benefits are astounding!

- Anti-depressant

- Fights anxiety

- Relieves stress

- Reduces pain
- Heals skin
- Cures infection
- Natural Deodorant
- Reduces fever
- Protects against cavities
- Helps the digestive system
- Great for aromatherapy
- Massage oil
- Helps with bug bite inflammation
- Anti biotic

Rosemary
Another herb, more benefits

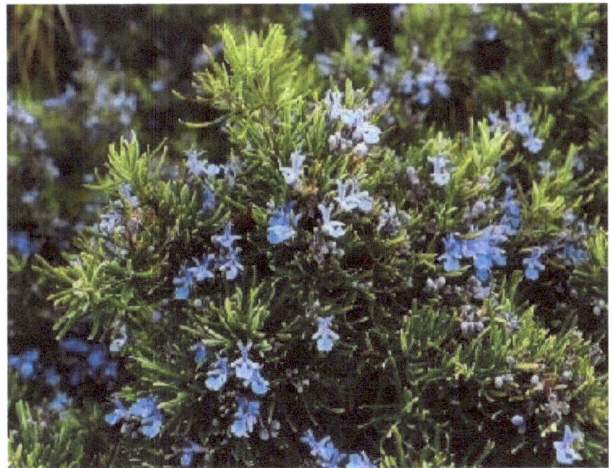

One of my favorites in the kitchen is quickly becoming one of my favorite oils too!

- Anti-aging

- Improves memory

- Promotes healthy kidneys

- Antibacterial

- Antidepressant

- Helps with migraines

- Improves blood flow

- Natural pain killer

- Mood enhancer
- Boosts immune system
- Relieves menstrual cramps
- Promotes respiratory health
- Natural mouthwash
- Promotes good hair health
- Boosts energy
- Antiviral
- Antiseptic

Chamomile
It's not just a tea

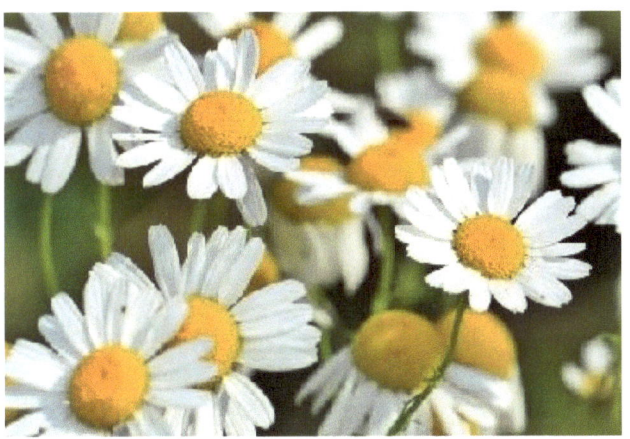

I love the tea, but I love the oil even more.

- Fights anxiety and depression
- Promotes healthy sleep
- Promotes good heart health
- Reduces nausea
- Calming
- Fights acne
- Helps skin conditions
- Reduces signs of aging
- High source of antioxidants

- Improves digestion
- Relieves congestion
- Helps fight cancer
- Pain reducer
- Decreases irritability

Jasmine

It sounds as pretty as it smells.

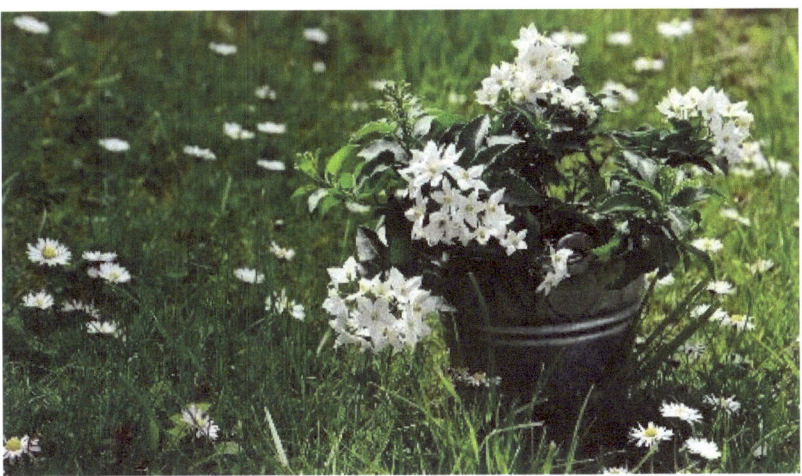

This one is just great and the benefits speak for themselves.

- Fights depression and anxiety

- Increases arousal

- Fights insomnia

- Improves immune system

- Fights infection

- Decreases symptoms of menopause

- Prevents PMS symptoms

- Reduces respiratory infections

- Boosts concentration
- Helps fade scarring
- Relaxes muscle spasm
- Antiseptic
- Reduces snoring
- Promotes lactation in mothers
- Helps protect uterus from tumors
- Facilitates birthing process
- Reduces labor pains in women
- Fights eczema
- Reduces nervousness
- Increases fertility

Orange
Back to the citrus

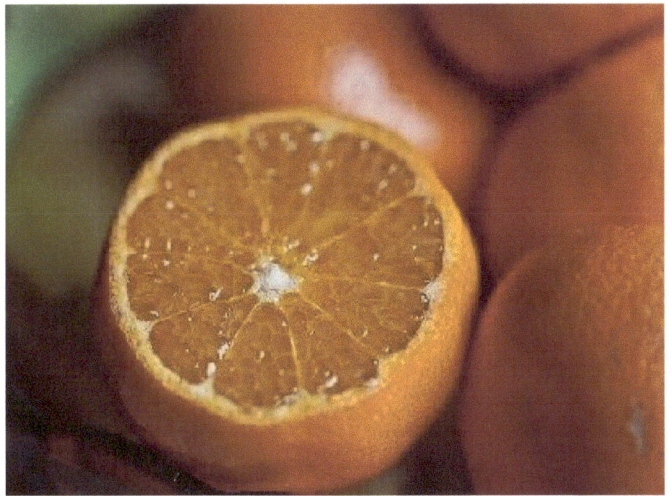

Orange is my go to at all times, literally all times.

- Boosts immune system
- Antibacterial
- Kitchen cleaner
- Boosts circulation
- Anti-inflammatory
- Reduces pain
- Boosts mood
- Promotes healthy digestion

- Anti-cancer benefits
- Reduces blood pressure and protects heart
- Gets rid of ants
- Treats constipation
- Relaxes muscles
- Fights anxiety
- Antidepressant
- Cures acne
- Disinfectant

Grapefruit
Citrus, citrus, citrus.

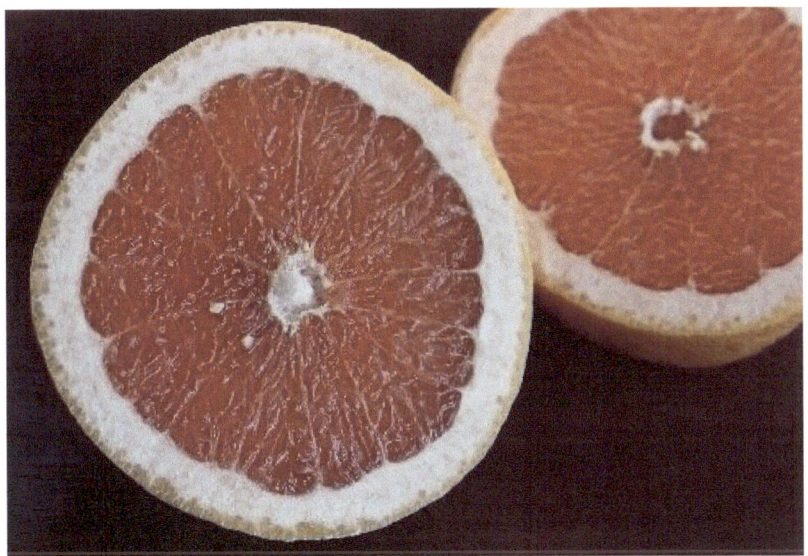

Can you tell I love the citrus oils?

- Weight loss booster
- Antibacterial
- Candida Killer
- Reduces stress
- Cures hangovers
- Stops bad cravings

- Natural air freshener
- Boosts circulation
- Diminishes cellulite
- Relieves menstrual cramps
- Treats acne and blemishes
- Disinfectant

Cypress
Oils, oils, and more oils.

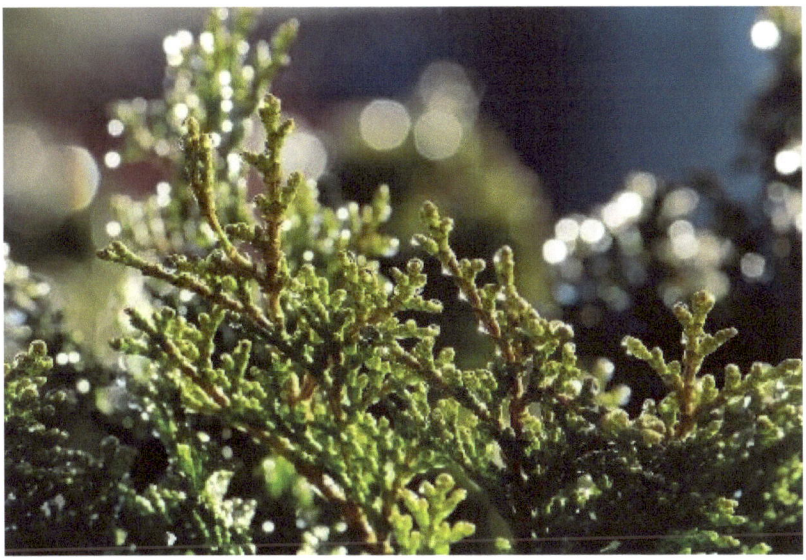

Seriously, with all these benefits, I literally just want to spend hundreds of dollars so I can have all of these oils at once.

- Cures spasms

- Promotes blood clotting

- Reduces heavy menstruation

- Ensures healthy liver

- Improves lung efficiency

- Causes sweating to help release toxins

- Sedative
- Helps treat both internal and external wounds

Thieves
No, not the kind of people who steal stuff

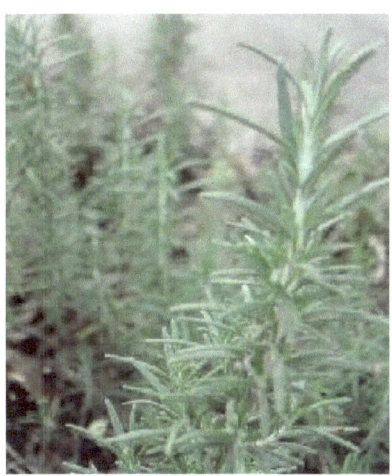

The ultimate immune booster, but it does more!

- Supports immune system

- Great for cleaning

- Support oral health

- Aids oral discomfort

- Prevents infection

- Promotes healing

- Reduces sore throat

- Relieves headache

- Helps with bronchitis

- Prevents and treats gum disease
- Gets rid of mold
- Pain relief
- Helps get rid of cold sores
- Repels insects
- Reduces the chances of cavities

Cloves
The list never ends!

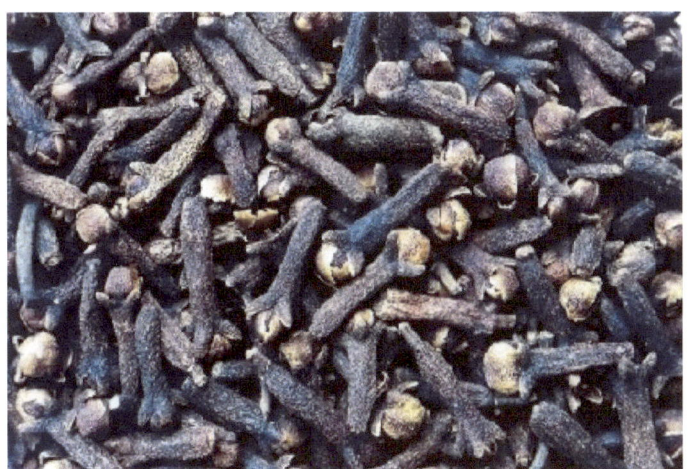

And let the benefits continue...

- Reduces joint pain

- Reduces symptoms of cough or cold

- Boosts the immune system

- Soothes arthritis

- Helps reduce varicose veins

- Improves blood circulation

- Reduces depression and anxiety

- Reduces headaches

- Stress reducer

- Reduce toothaches
- Soothes nausea
- Reduces bloating
- Reduces congestion
- Helps with achy muscles
- Helps with athlete's foot

Ginger
Another household item gone oil

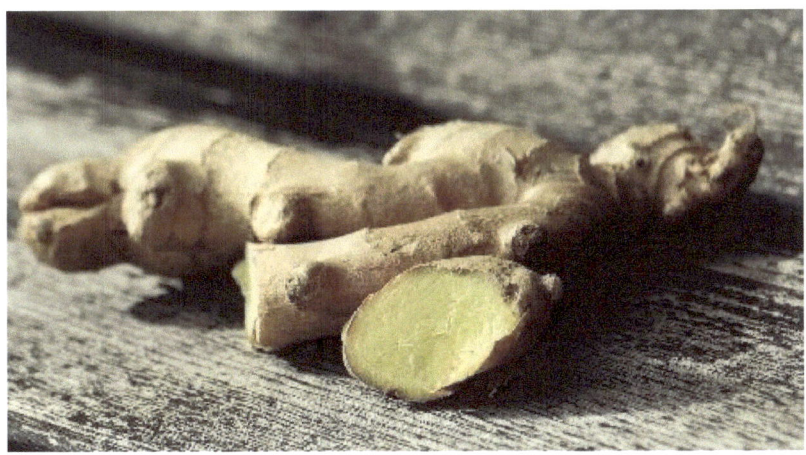

The list seriously never ends!

- Reduces nausea

- Helps with motion sickness

- Soothes muscle aches

- Reduces muscle spasms and cramps

- Increases circulation

- Soothes sore throat

- Reduces stress

- Promotes heart health

- Reduces morning sickness

- Prevents gas and bloating

- Anti-cancer
- Reduces pain and inflammation
- Antibiotic
- Cold and flu prevention
- Migraine relief

Geranium
Another day, another oil

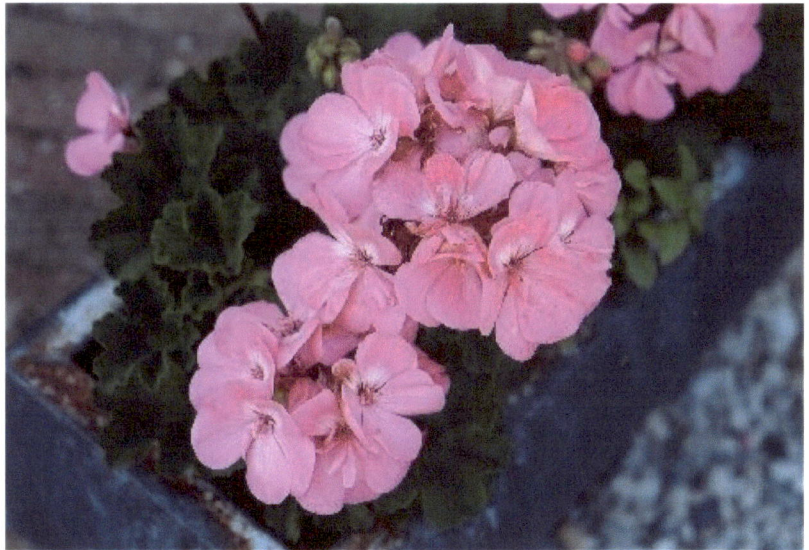

This one has found a spot in my garden and my home!

- Reduces stress and anxiety

- Promotes healthy skin

- Balances out hormones

- Reduces allergies

- Cancer-killing properties

- Speeds wound healing
- Insect repellent
- Supports adrenal fiction
- Eases hemorrhoid pain
- Helps cure Urinary tract infections
- Improves brain clarity and concentration
- Decreases blood sugar problems
- Improves hair and scalp health
- Helps heal cold sores
- Anti-fungal

Basil
The herbs are taking over!

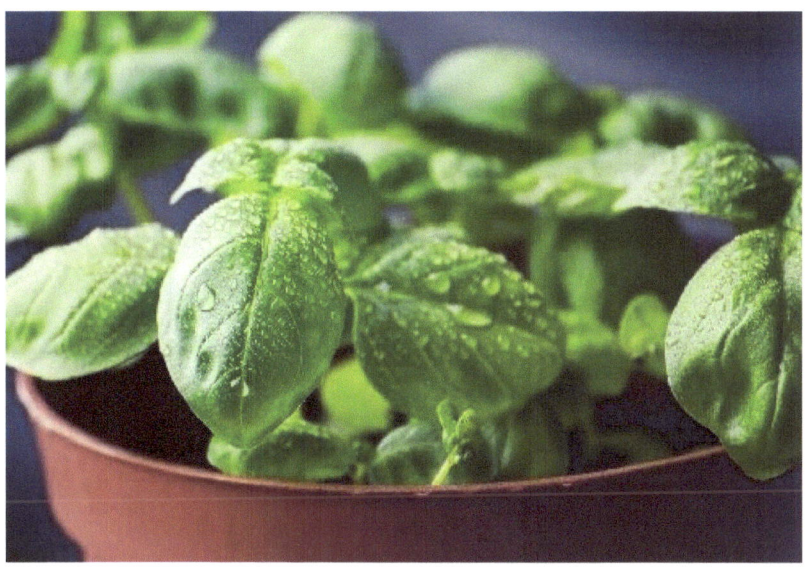

Not just for food, but for health too.

- Contains disease fighting antioxidants
- Anti-inflammatory
- Fights cancer
- Antibacterial
- Antidepressant

- Promotes cardiovascular health
- Supports liver function
- Natural aphrodisiac
- Helps protect from diabetes
- Insect repellant
- Assists digestion
- Improves mental clarity when applied to brain stem and spine
- Migraine relief

Cedarwood
We're getting pretty outdoorsy here!

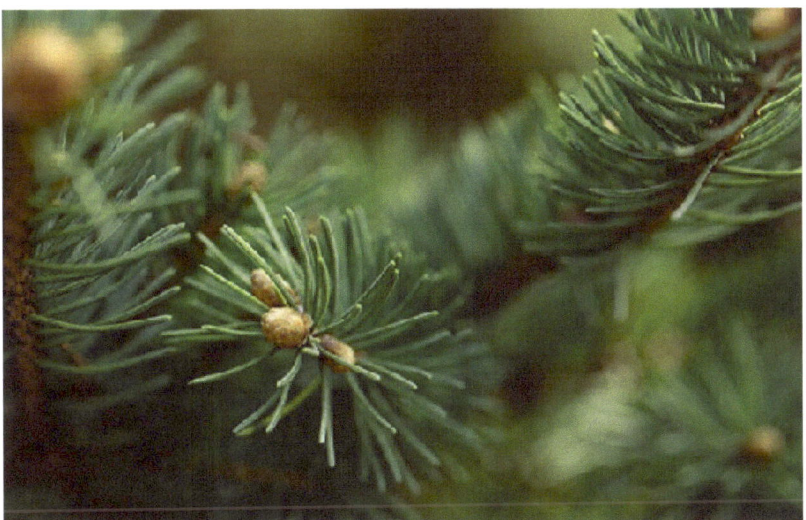

My favorite woodsy scent of all time.

- Reduces hair loss

- Reduces eczema

- Reduces dry scalp

- Antiseptic

- Reduces arthritis

- Natural deodorizer

- Relieves spasmodic conditions
- Tightens muscles
- Promotes healthy sleep habits
- Fights acne
- Insect repellant
- Pain relief
- Helps heal minor wounds
- Anti-fungal

Patchouli
The blends are coming soon I promise!

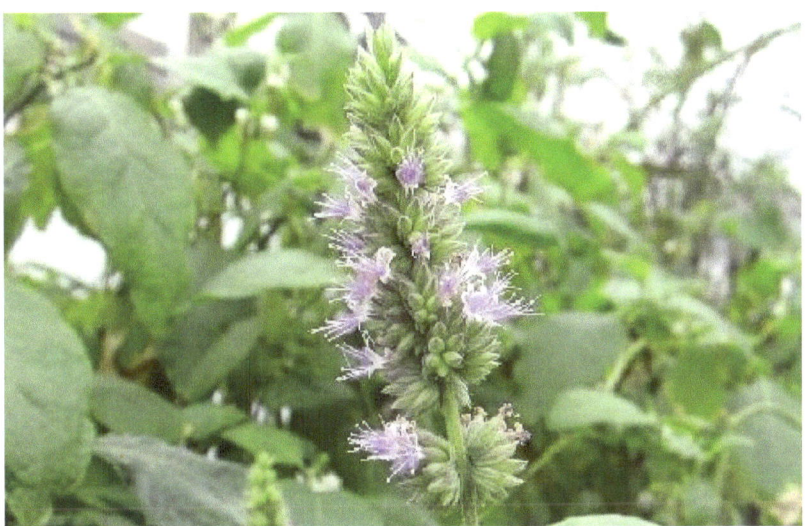

Do you feel your health getting better page by page? I know I do!

- Helps heal wounds

- Aromatherapy

- Promotes healthy skin

- Insect repellant

- Natural deodorant

- Good massage oil

- Antidepressant
- Anti-inflammatory
- Prevents infection
- Stimulates hormones
- Helps metabolic system
- Minimizes scars
- Strengthens hair
- Calming
- Promotes good balance
- Respiratory support

Spearmint
Minty fresh

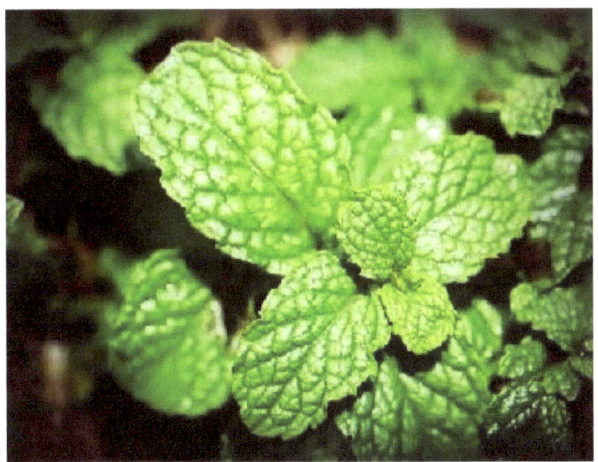

Who doesn't love some minty freshness?

- Helps treat asthma

- Relaxes nerves and muscles

- Improves concentration

- Mosquito repellant

- Promotes good blood circulation

- Headache relief

- Stress relief

- Antiseptic

- Provides relief from menstrual cramps

- Aids proper organ function

Fennel
Another kitchen fresh item

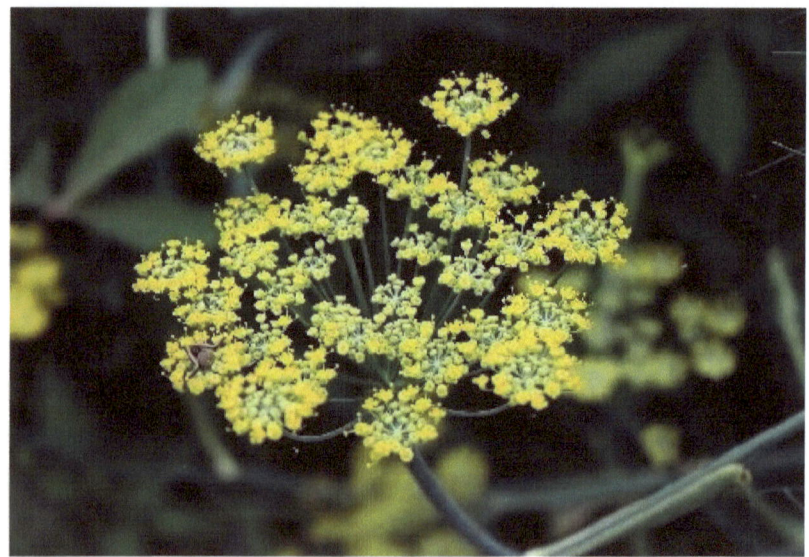

From the cutting board to your essential oil bottle.

- Promotes healthy metabolism

- Promotes healthy liver function

- Promotes healthy blood circulation

- Fights sweet tooth craving

- Helps with digestion

- Promotes healthy respiratory tract

- Freshens breath

- Soothes stomach pains

- Aids weight loss

- Relieves gas and constipation

- Heals wounds

- Reduces and prevents gut spasms

- Antibiotic

- Helps cure Urinary tract infection

Thyme
More herbs saving the day!

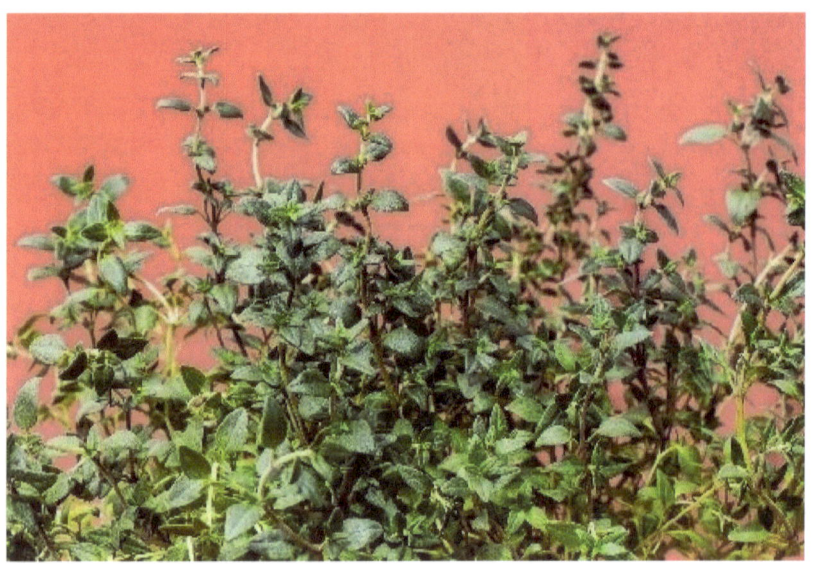

Thyme is another favorite in the kitchen, but I love it even more as an oil.

- Treats respiratory conditions
- Kills bacteria
- Promotes skin health
- Promotes teeth health
- Increases blood circulation

- Reduces stress
- Reduces anxiety
- Balances hormones
- Shown to kill Breast Cancer Cells
- Treats fibroids
- Prevents formation of gas in stomach and intestines
- Diuretic
- Boosts memory and concentration
- Reduces cellulite
- Prevents hair loss
- Improves vision

Bring on the Blends!

I would never leave you without some amazing blends to try!

These blends are great to put in a spray bottle, put in a roller bottle, or stick into your diffuser!

My Favorite Allergy Blend

2 Drops of Lavender

2 Drops of Lemon

2 Drops of Peppermint

Sleeping Baby

7 Drops of Chamomile

5 Drops of Lavender

Stress No More

2 Drops of Lemon

4 Drops of Lavender

6 Drops of Clary Sage

Focus

6 Drops Rosemary

4 Drops Lemon

2 Drops Peppermint

Mood Boost

2 Drops Bergamot

2 Drops Lemon

2 Drops Orange

Peace out Congestion

3 Drops of Peppermint

2 Drops of Eucalyptus

2 Drops of Tea Tree oil

1 Drop of Lemon

Energy Boost

2 Drops of Peppermint

2 Drops of Orange

2 Drops of Grapefruit

Romance

2 Drops of Lavender

2 Drops of Patchouli

2 Drops of Geranium

2 Drops of Ylang Ylang

Fresh and Clean

2 Drops of Lavender

2 Drops of Lemon

1 Drop of Rosemary

Key Lime Pie

2 Drops of Lemon

3 Drops of Lime

Fresh Flowers

3 Drops of Jasmine

3 Drops of Ylang Ylang

2 Drops of Lavender

Island Breeze

4 Drops of Bergamot

4 Drops of Lime

Rise and Shine

3 Drops of Peppermint

2 Drops of Lemon

2 Drops of Orange

Nerve Pain Blend (best in roller bottle)

20 Drops of Basil

20 Drops of Lavender

20 Drops of Geranium

Fill the rest of bottle with coconut oil

Cough and Cold Blend

4 Drops of Tea Tree

4 Drops of Frankincense

4 Drops of Cedarwood

Cleanliness

3 Drops of Lime

3 Drops of Lemon

2 Drops of Lavender

2 Drops of Rosemary

Laser Focus

2 Drops of Vetiver

2 Drops of Lavender

Clarity

2 Drops of Peppermint

2 Drops of Frankincense

Gypsy

3 Drops of Grapefruit

2 Drops of Patchouli

The Ultimate Anxiety Blend

7 Drops of Basil

7 Drops of Bergamot

3 Drops of Peppermint

2 Drops of Lavender

1 Drop of Eucalyptus

Take me to The Beach

2 Drops of Lavender

2 Drops of Bergamot

1 Drop Rosemary

1 Drops Eucalyptus

Migraine Relief

3 Drops of Lemongrass

2 Drops of Peppermint

5 Drops of Lavender